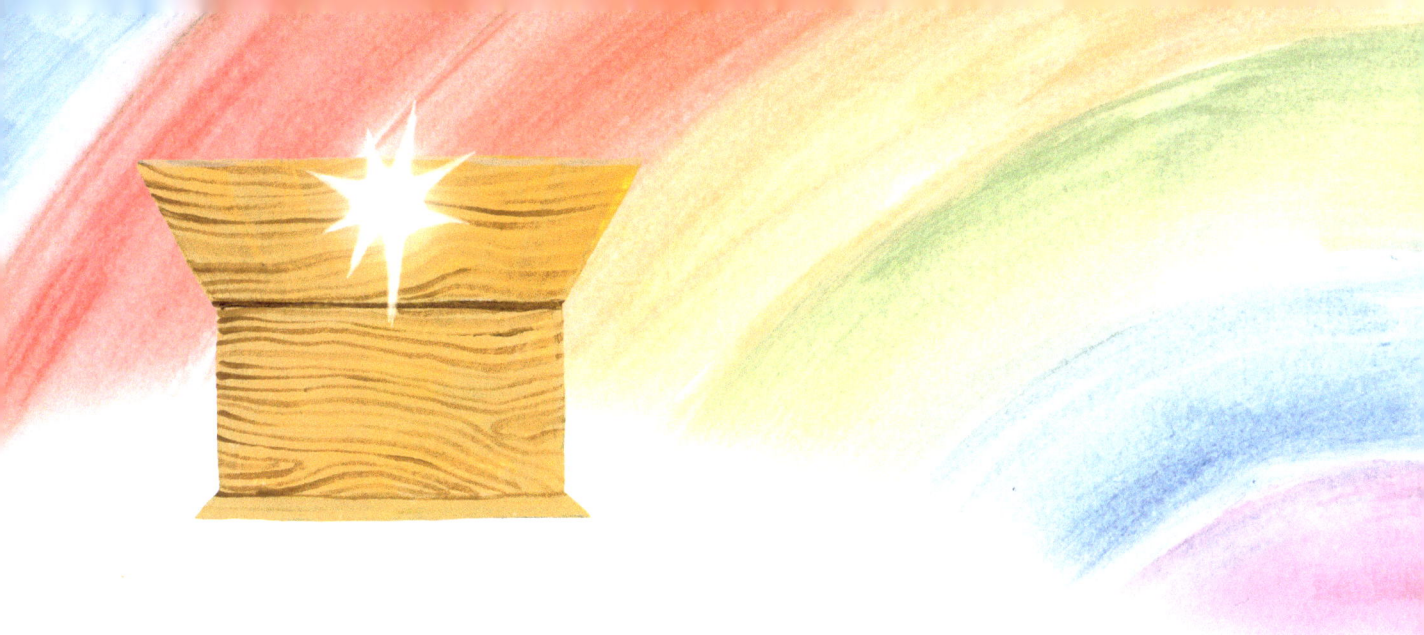

RAINBOW BABY

By

Jami-Leigh Sawyer, PhD
& Jude Milinovich

Illustrated by Sari Richter

ISBN 978-1-7774813-0-8

All rights are reserved.
Copyright ©2021 Jami-Leigh Sawyer

Cover artwork and illustrations by Sari Richter

For all content, photographs, etc. that contain specific brand names or brand products, these are copyrighted and/or trademarked by the respective companies and/or organizations, unless otherwise specified.

This book, or parts thereof, may not be reproduced in any form, stored in or introduced into a retrieval system, or transmitted in any form or by any means (electronic, mechanical, photocopying, recording or otherwise), without written permission of the copyright holder.

For information: www.jamileighsawyer.com

First edition
Published in Canada

This is a work of fiction. Names, characters, places, and incidents are either the product of the author's imagination or are used fictitiously, and any resemblance to business establishments, events, locales, or actual persons, living or dead, is entirely coincidental.

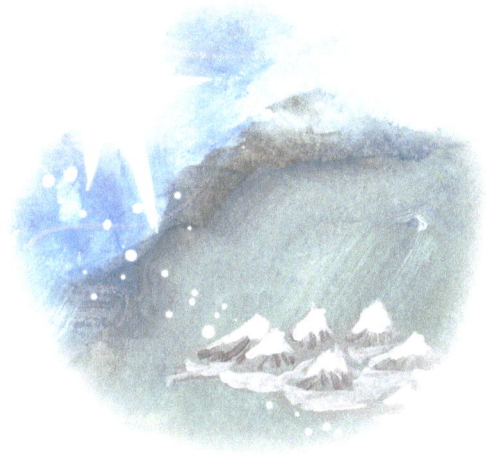

This book is dedicated to miracle Myles, rainbow Jude, and pot of gold Everly Hope.

It is also devoted to every person navigating the grief of losing a child. Whether you are with or without a rainbow after the storm, we honour you deeply.

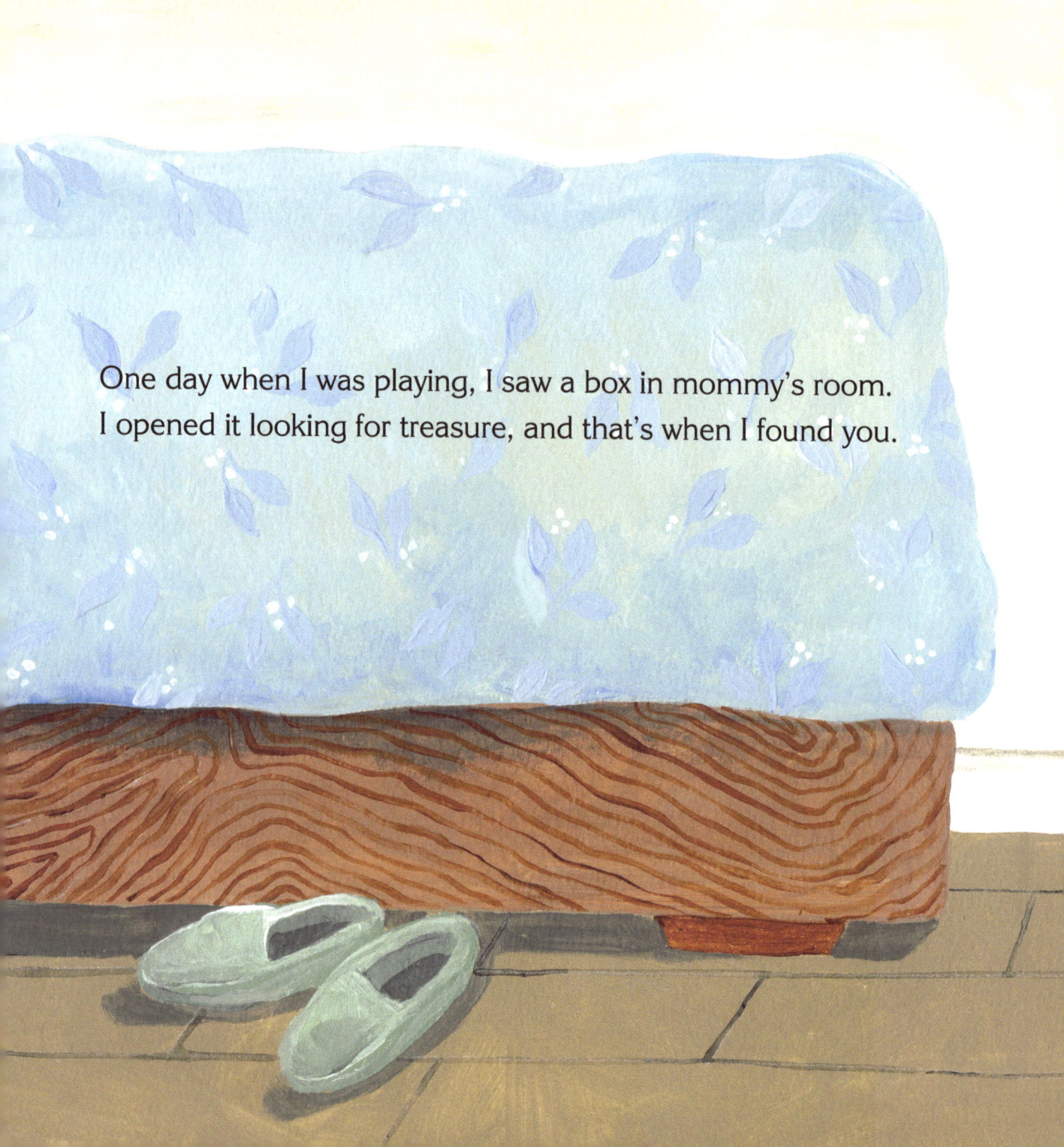

One day when I was playing, I saw a box in mommy's room. I opened it looking for treasure, and that's when I found you.

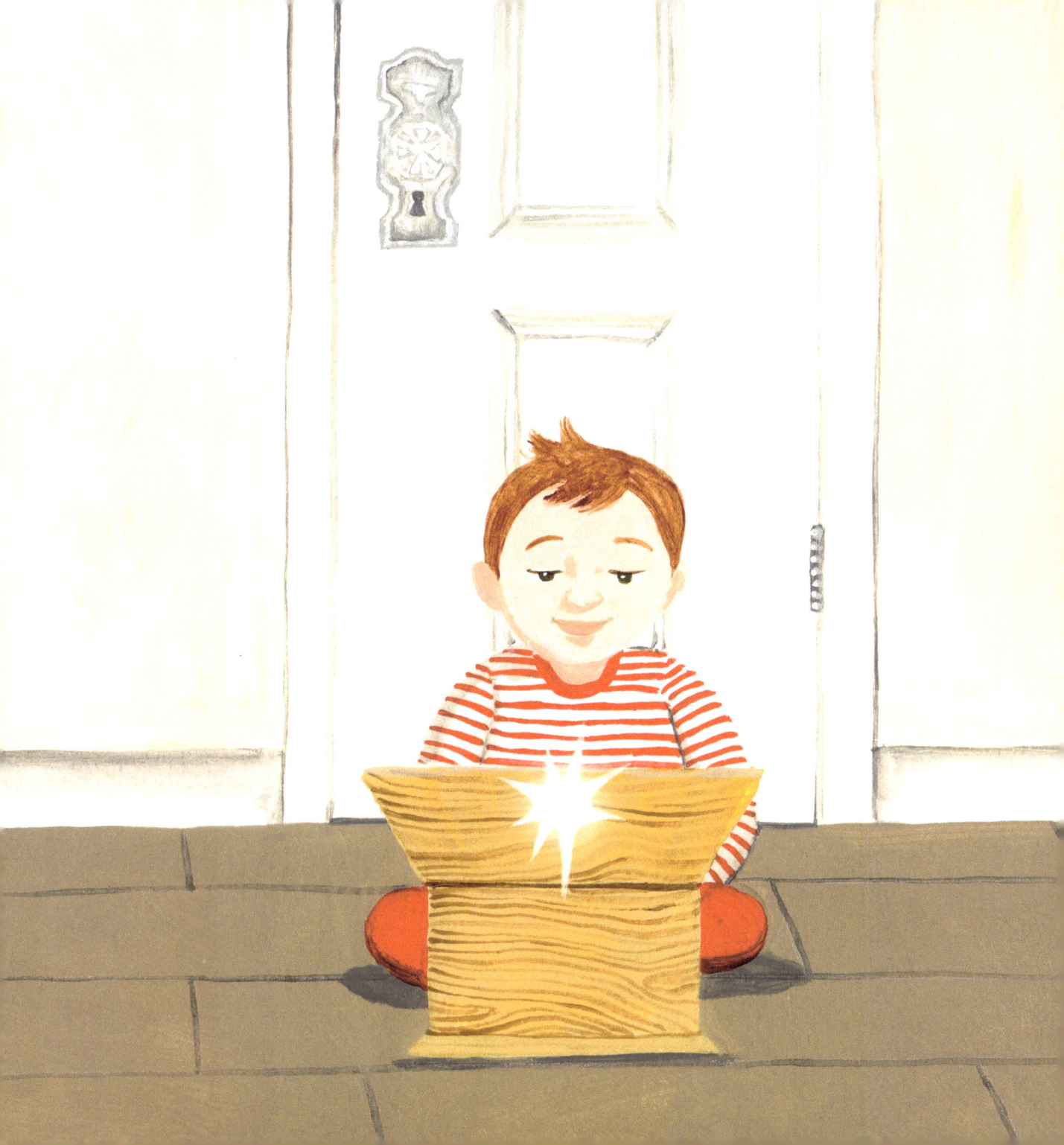

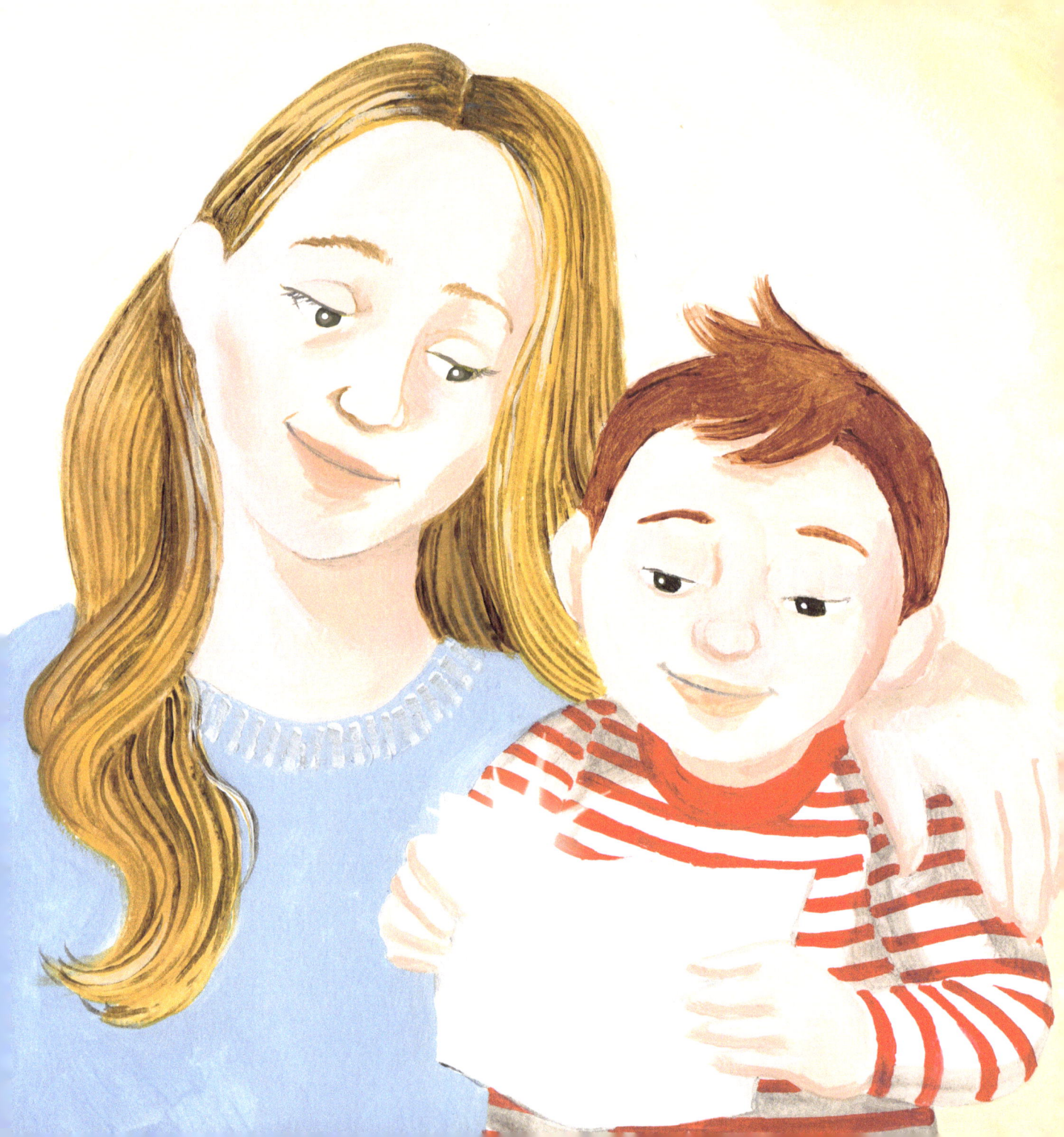

You looked so small in your picture,
but I could surely see you there,
And from the look on mommy's face,
I could see how much she cares.

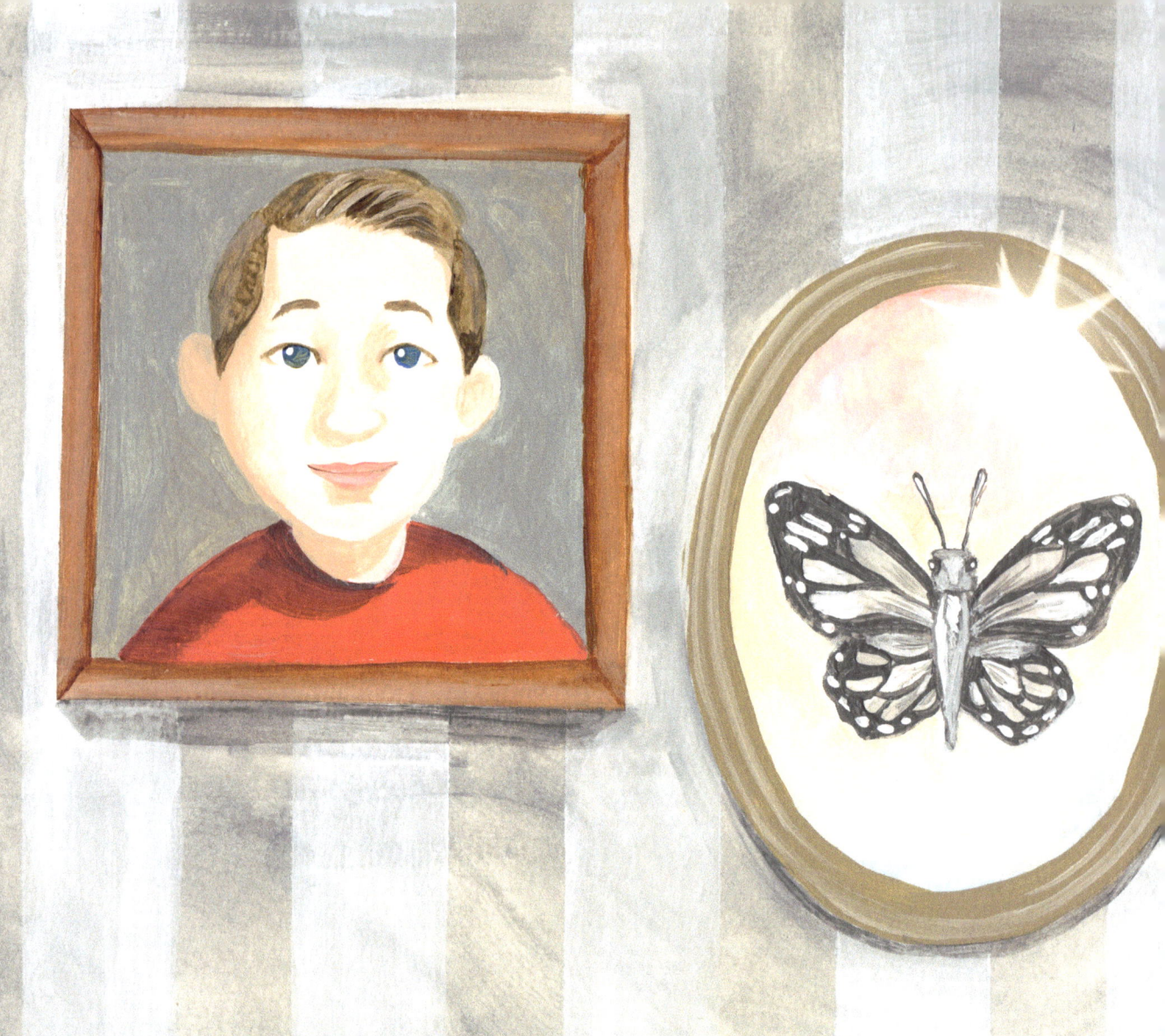

Your name and life are never hidden. There's a frame upon the wall,
Tucked beside mine and the others, so mommy can see us all.

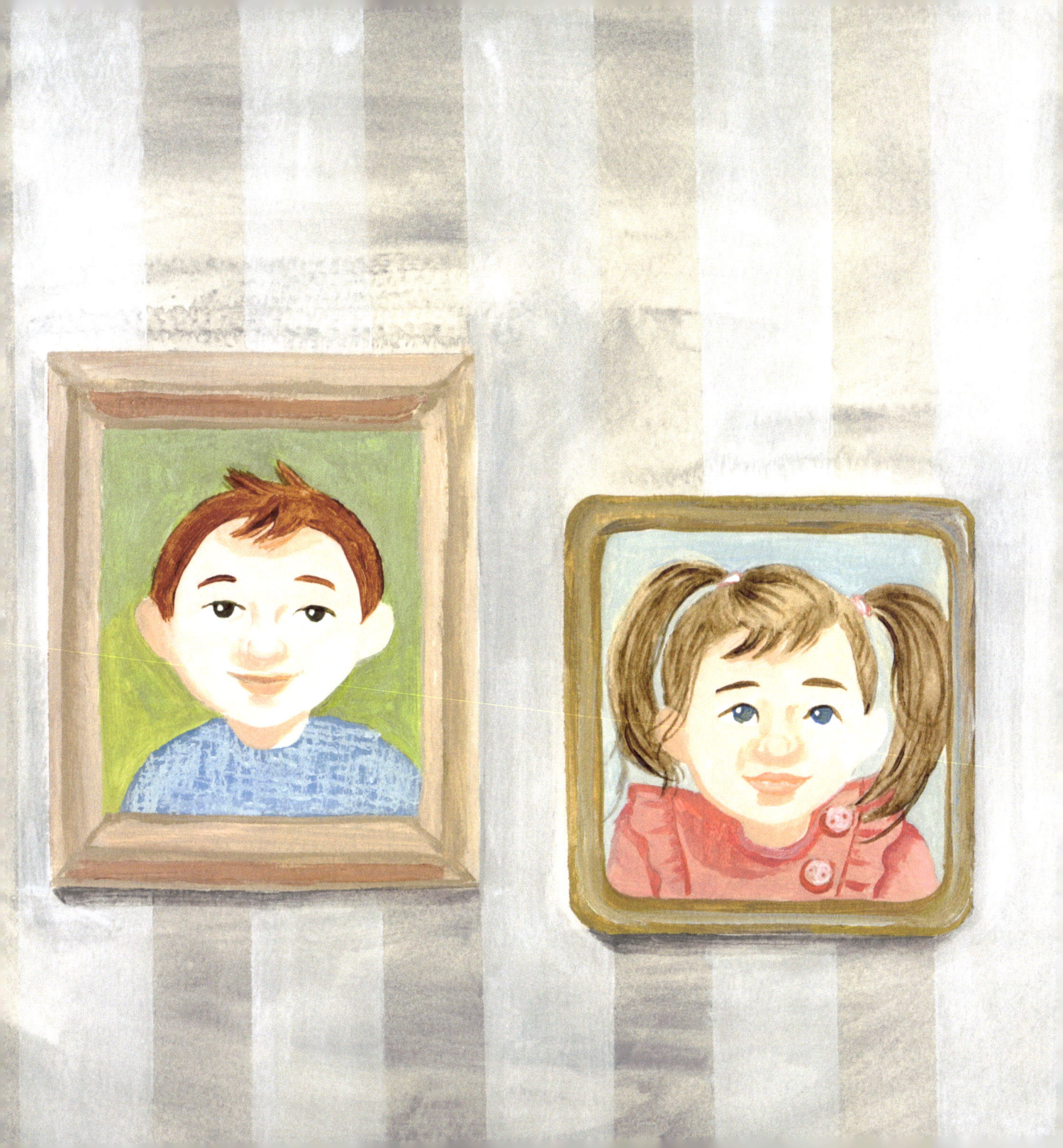

Sometimes in the night I see you. We play trucks, drink tea, and dance. We talk about the fun we would have had together, if you'd only had the chance.

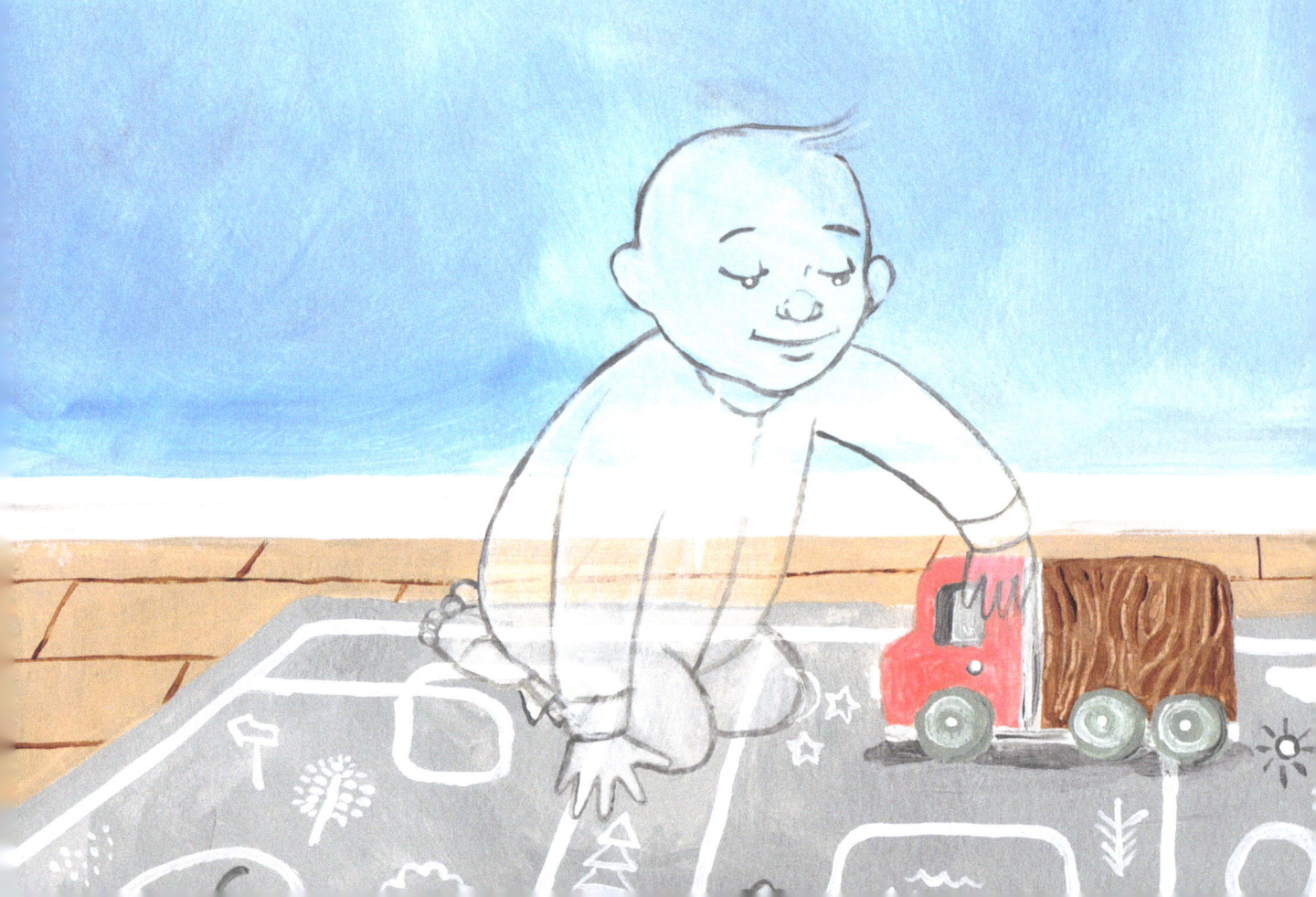

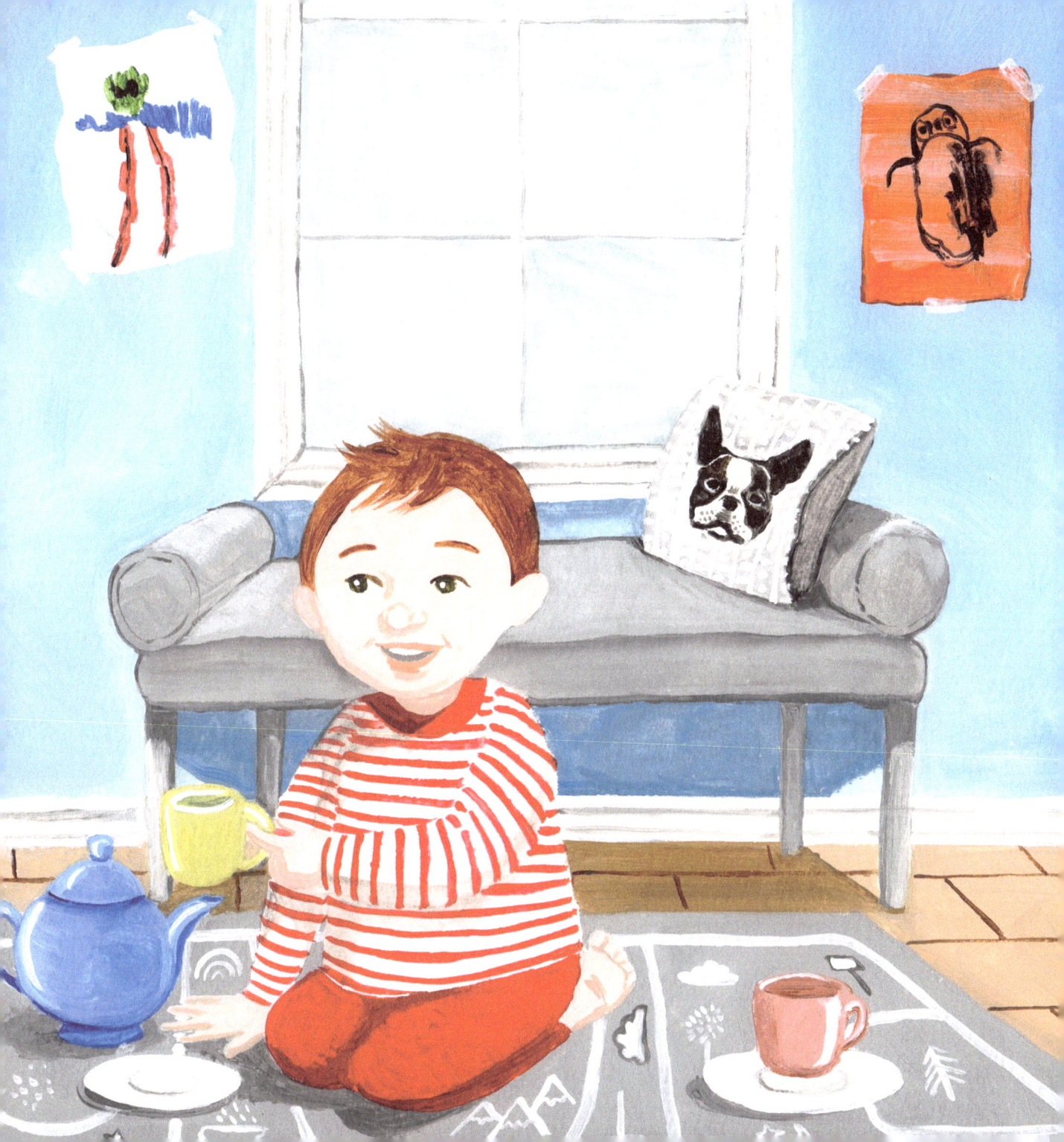

I am the rainbow baby that now walks this side of earth,
But you're the shining light that held my hand until my birth.

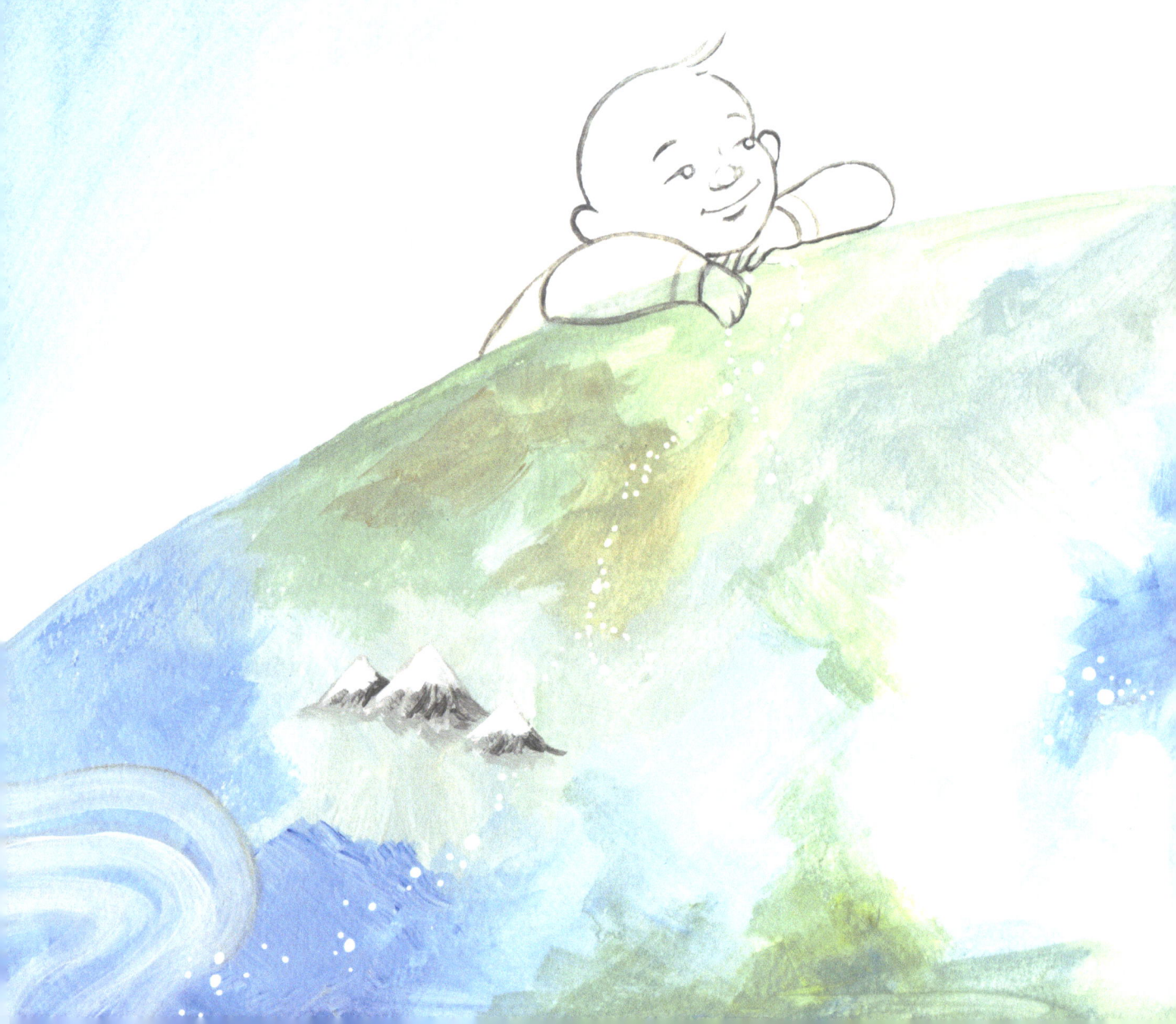

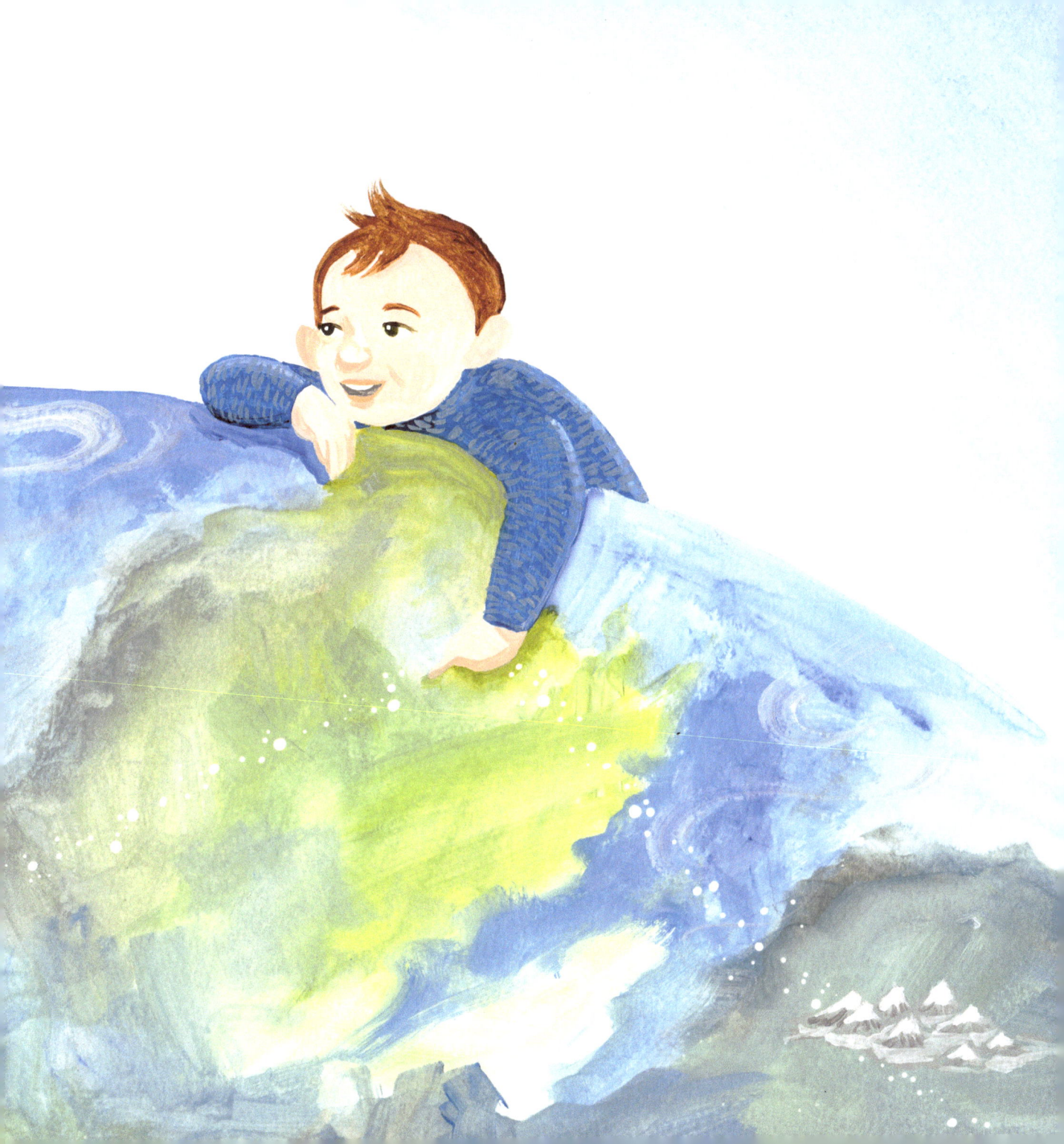

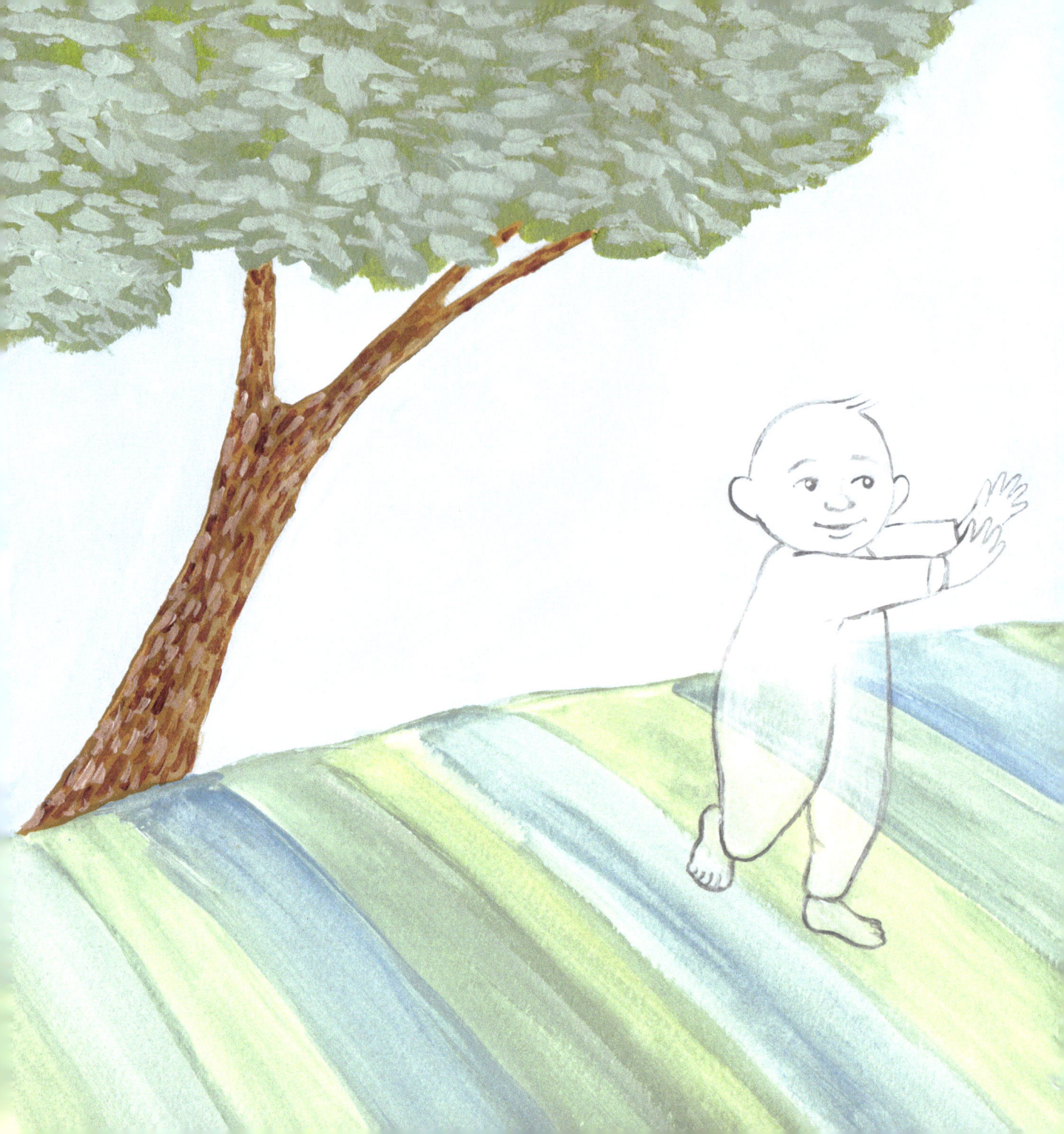

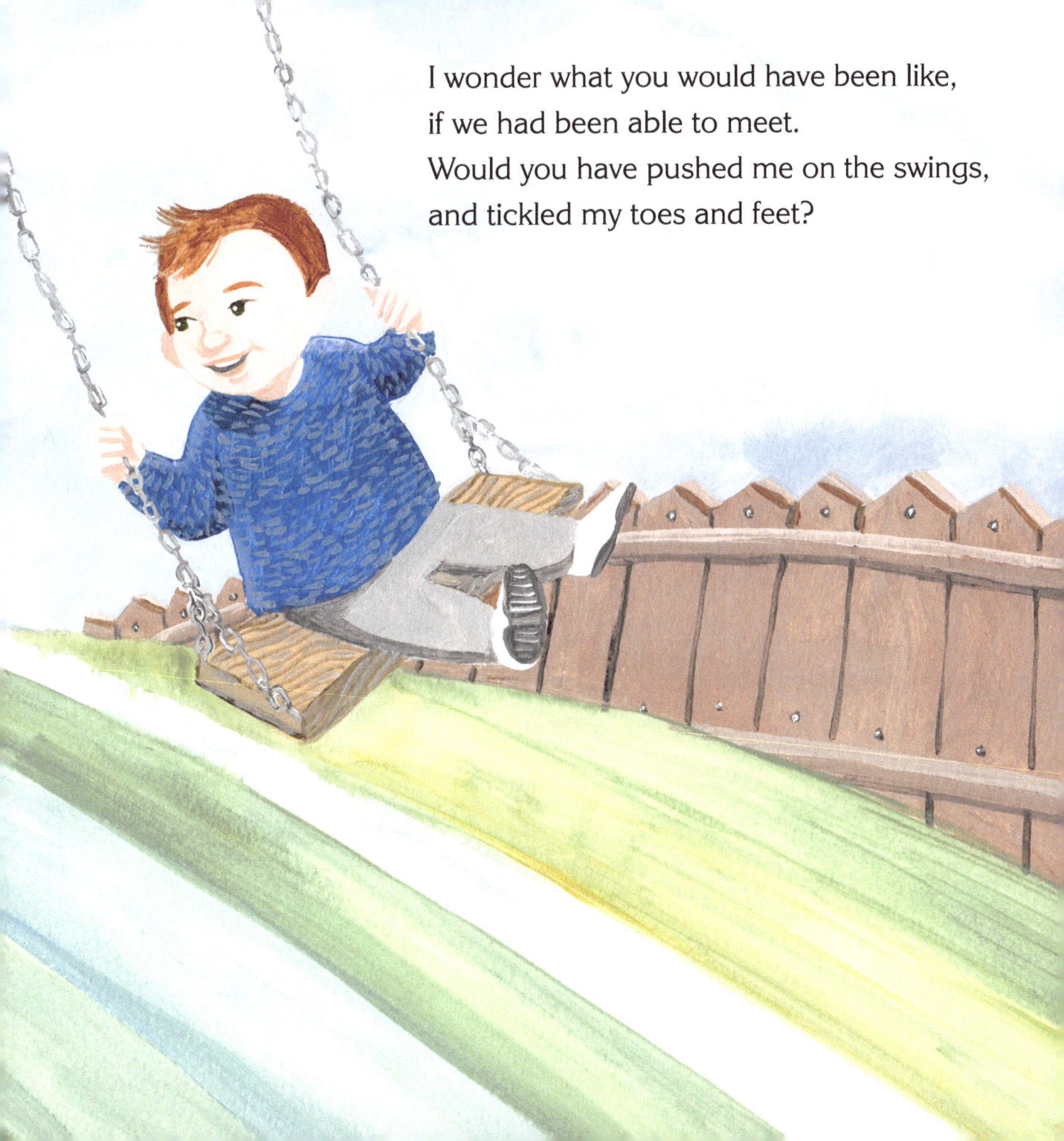

I wonder what you would have been like,
if we had been able to meet.
Would you have pushed me on the swings,
and tickled my toes and feet?

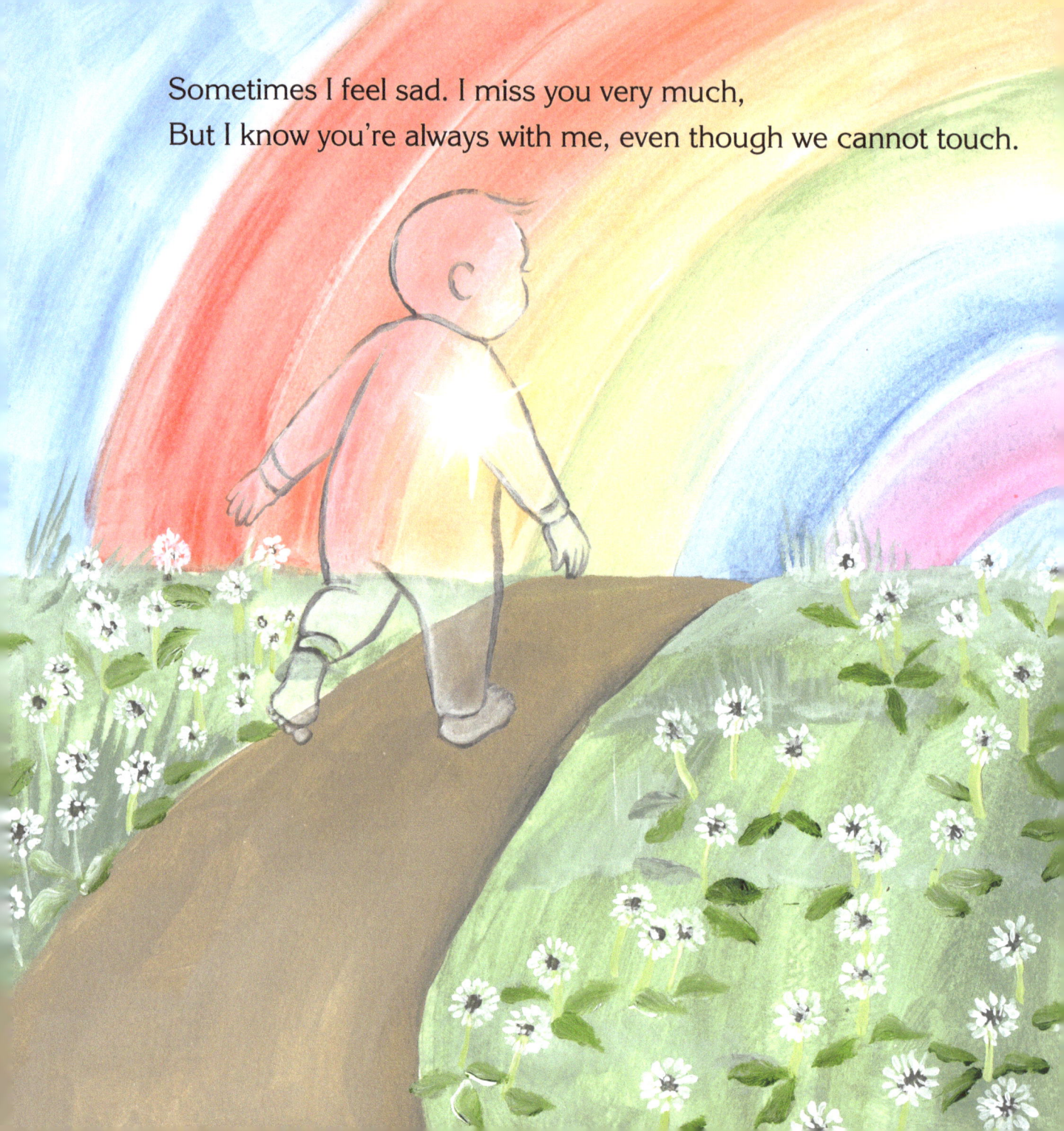
Sometimes I feel sad. I miss you very much,
But I know you're always with me, even though we cannot touch.

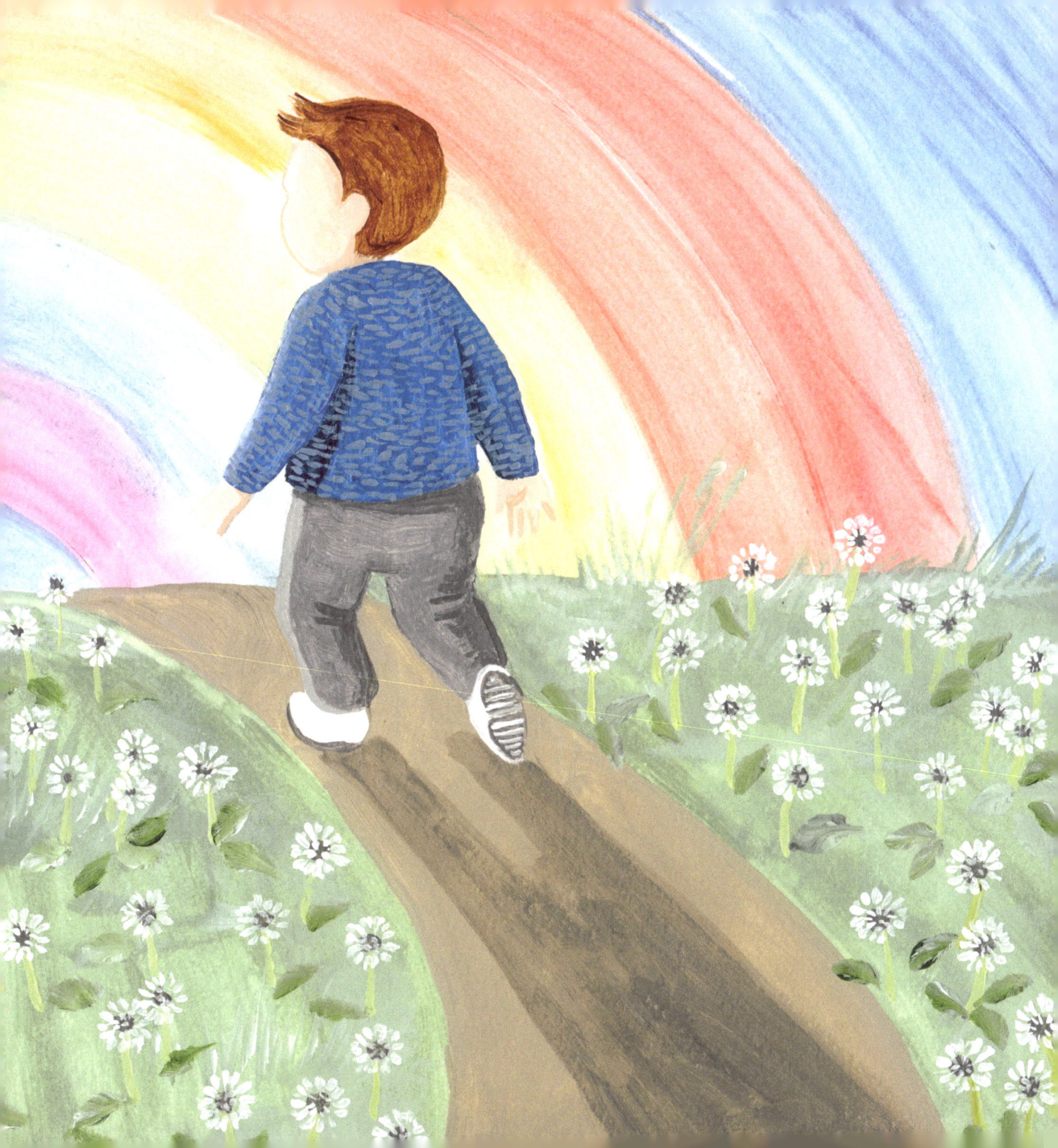

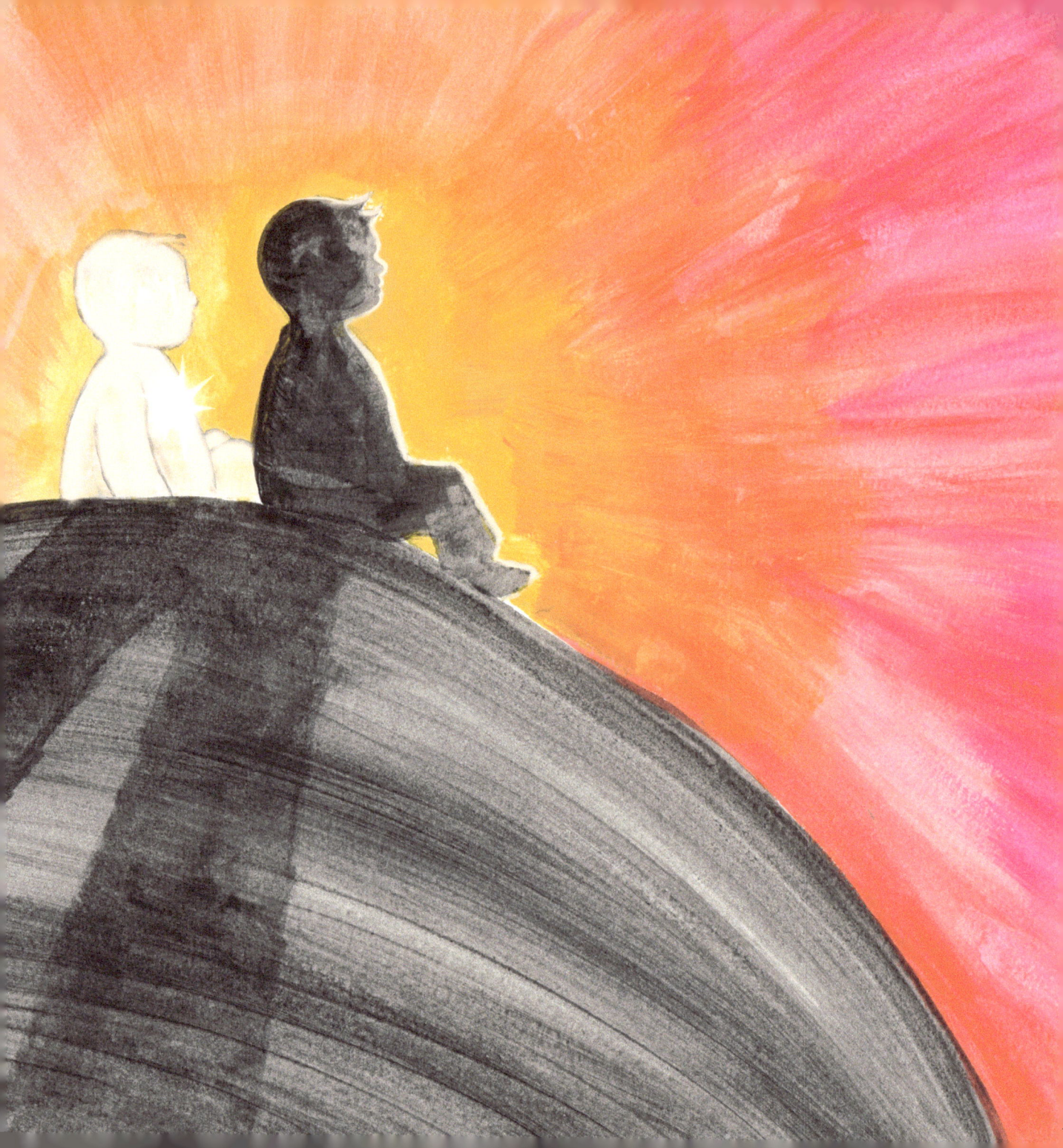

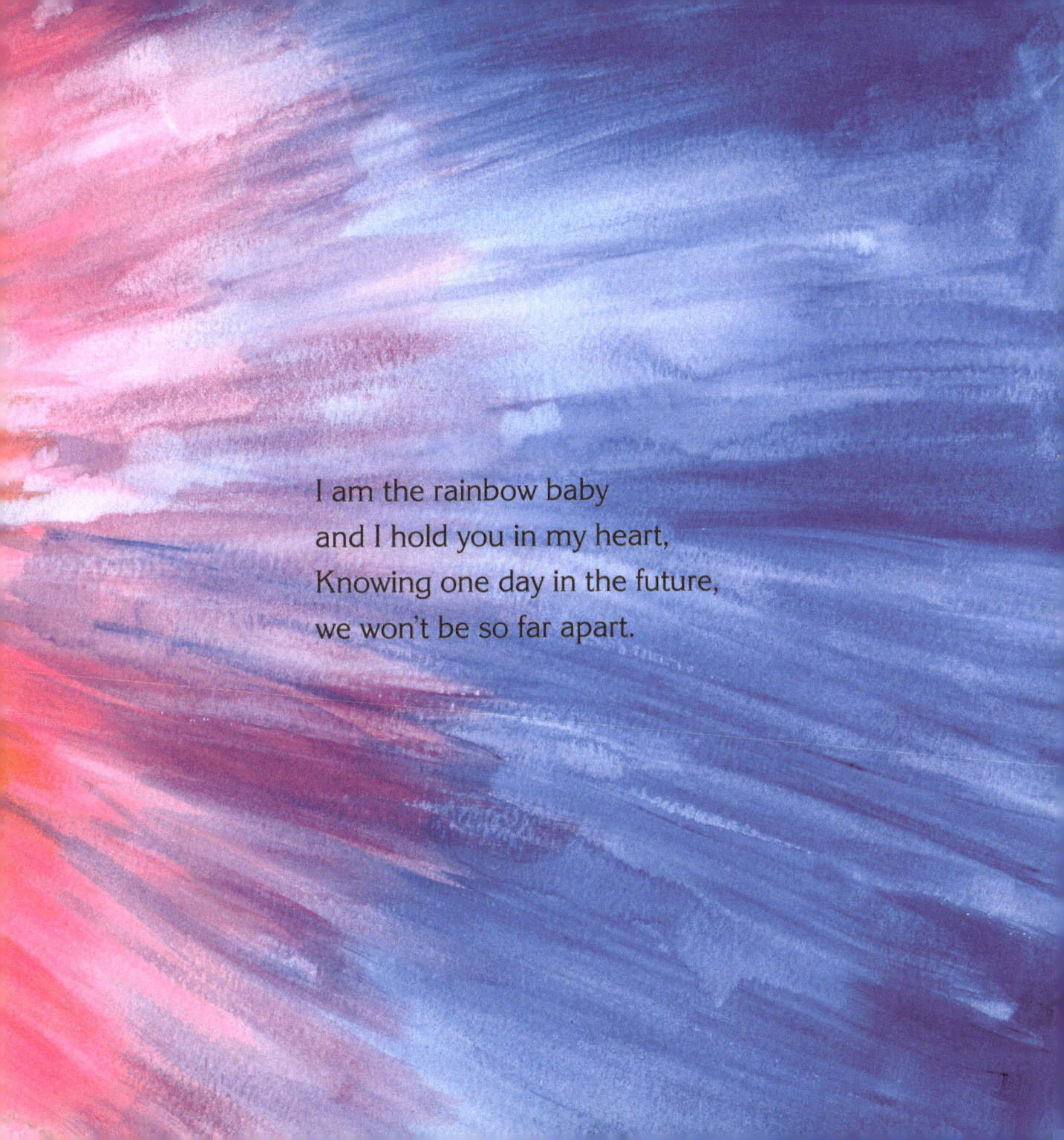

I am the rainbow baby
and I hold you in my heart,
Knowing one day in the future,
we won't be so far apart.

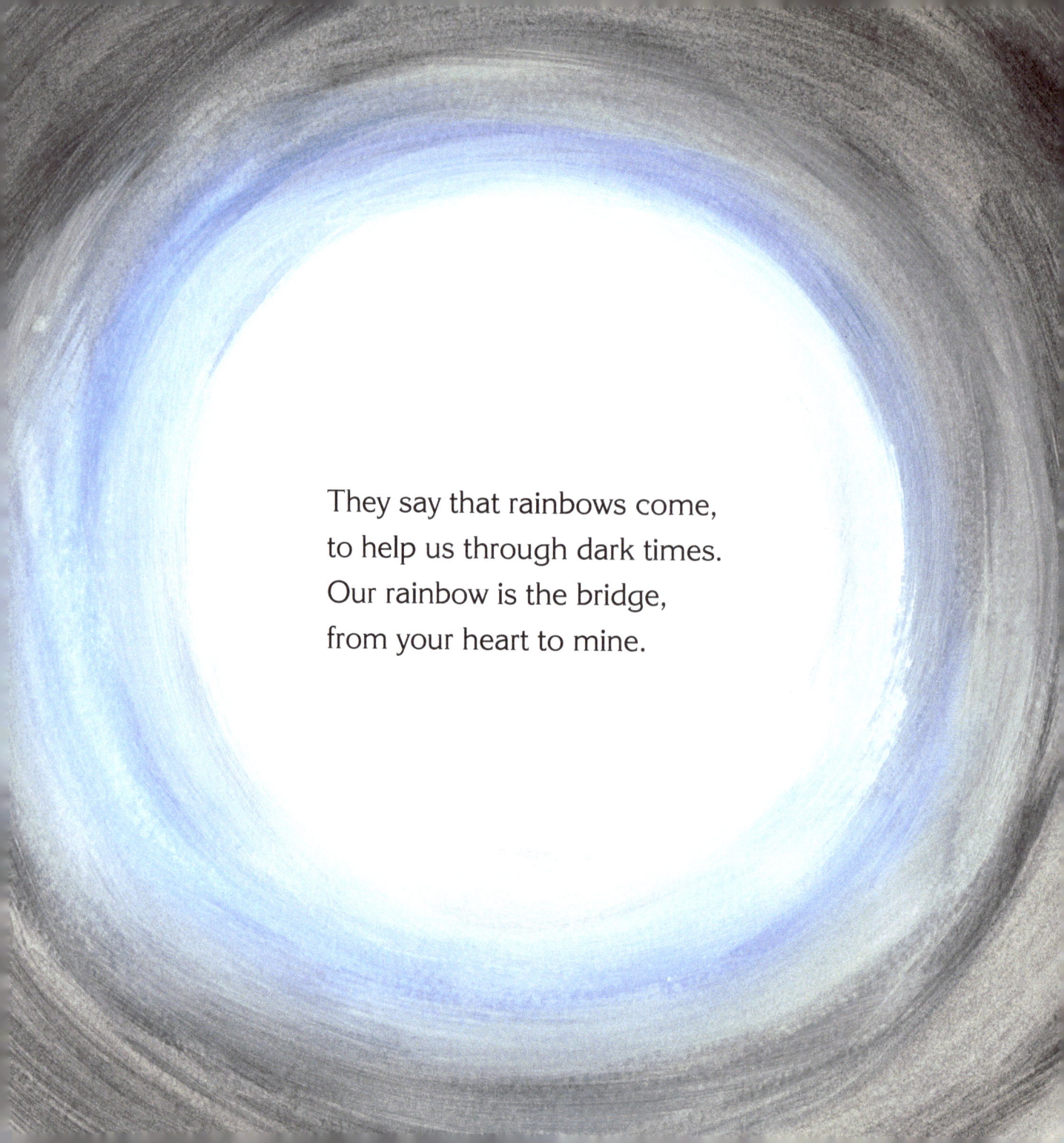

They say that rainbows come,
to help us through dark times.
Our rainbow is the bridge,
from your heart to mine.

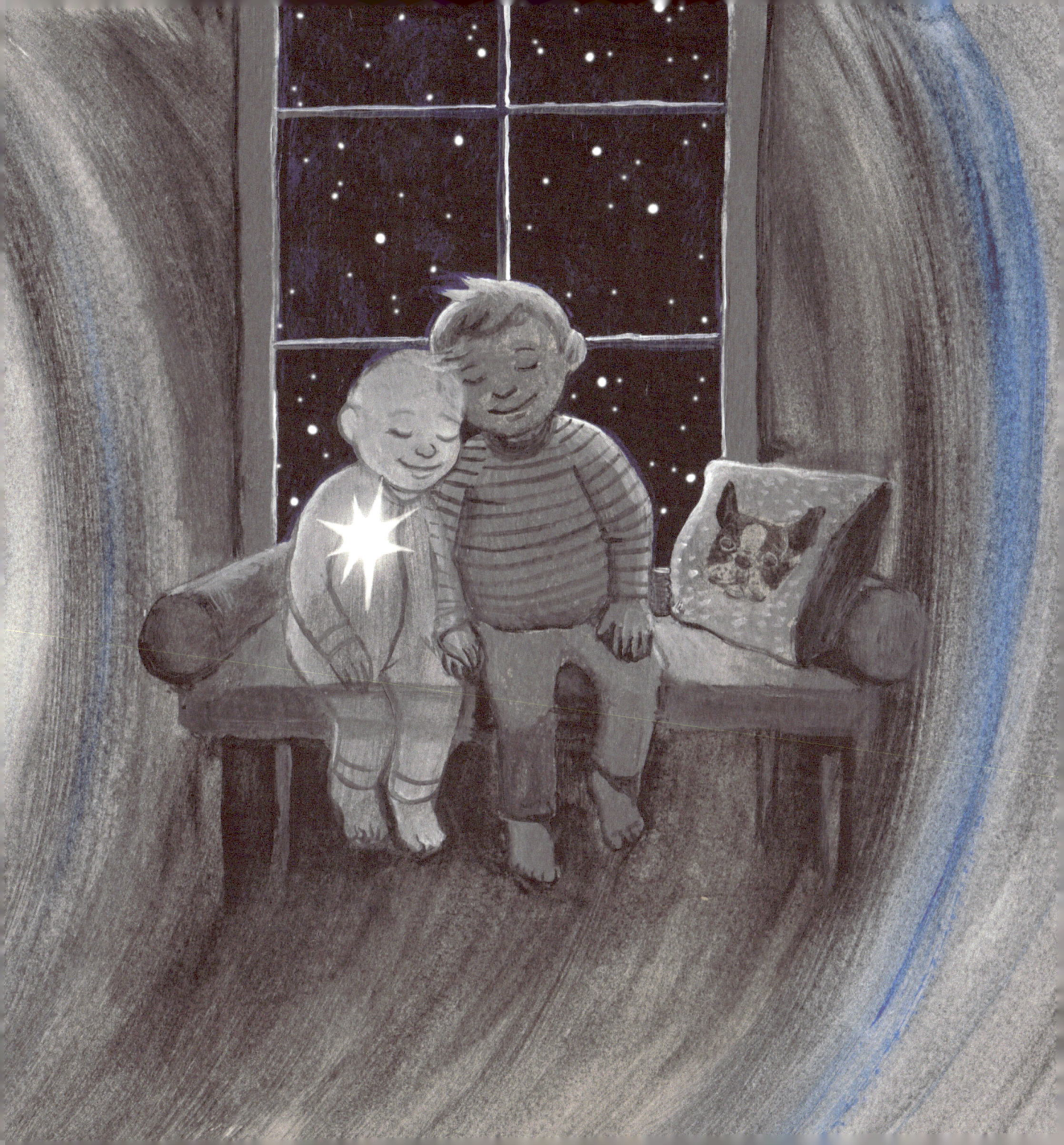

Jami-Leigh Sawyer, PhD

Jami-Leigh wrote Rainbow Baby using stories Jude shared of the twin siblings the family lost due to miscarriage. As a counsellor, she works to support individuals and couples on their journey to conceive. It is her "heart work" to support those who have experienced grief and loss along the way.

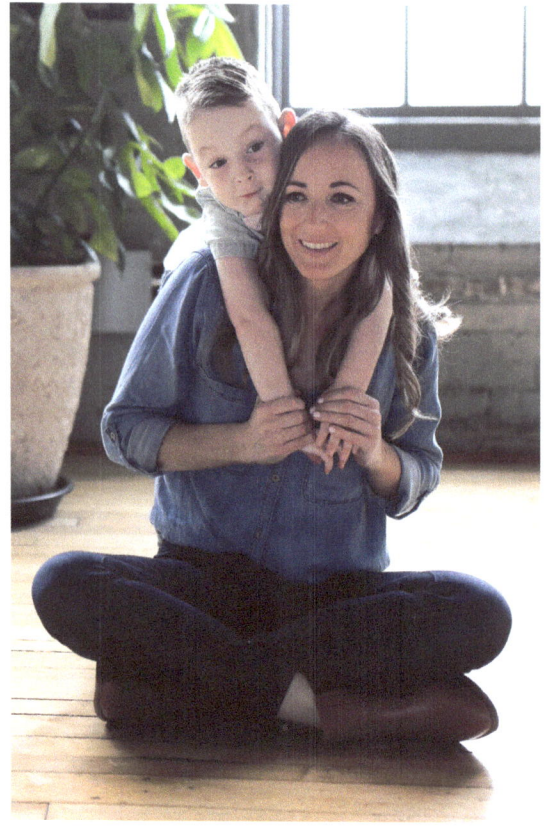

Jude Milinovich

As a young child, Jude is an artistic, curious, and sensitive boy with wisdom beyond his years. He enjoys playing outside, spending time with friends, and most of all playing with his brother and sister.

www.ingramcontent.com/pod-product-compliance
Lightning Source LLC
Chambersburg PA
CBHW041703160426
43209CB00017B/1732